25 Myths About Breastfeeding

By Lyria Haven

ISBN: 9798863881225

CONTENTS

CONTENTS

INTRODUCTION

Hey Mom, First off, congrats on this incredible journey! I'm Lyria Haven, and I've been in your shoes. I'm your go-to gal for everything from breastfeeding and baby care, to introducing those first bites of solid food and the eventual weaning process. I've got five awesome kiddos of my own. And just like you, I had to navigate through the ups and downs of motherhood – and that includes the challenges of breastfeeding. It feels like everyone has an opinion, right? From myths to "helpful" advice from well-meaning folks, it can get overwhelming.

But guess what?

Mother Nature's pretty smart. So, driven by my own experiences and the desire to support moms like you, I dived deep into learning all about it. I've spent over 200 hours training in various schools, and I've clocked in a whopping 800 hours working hands-on with moms. It's been a fulfilling journey; 95% of the moms I've advised are now happily breastfeeding their little ones. This guide? It's my way of sharing the real deal with you. I've debunked some age-old myths that get passed down through generations. Some of this stuff might sound familiar, but a lot of it's more like old wives' tales than facts. But don't worry, I've got your back! Science and medicine have given us a lot of answers. By the end of our time together, you'll see breastfeeding in a new light.

Think of it as a natural, chill process. You'll also get why there's no need to rush with stuff like water, "grown-up" food, and the whole debate on pacifiers

BREASTFEEDING IS COMPLICATED, INCONVENIENT, AND FULL OF PROBLEMS

There's nothing more straightforward, natural, and comfy than organized breastfeeding. The trick is to get prepped for it. Books, magazines, movies – they're all cool. But there's something magic about learning firsthand from someone who's been there – a mentor, a guide, a mom who's breastfed her kiddo for ages and genuinely enjoyed every moment. The world might make you think that there's some secret formula to breastfeeding. Spoiler alert: there isn't.

Like any skill, it just needs patience, practice, and a touch of guidance. Remember that each journey is unique. What works for one mom might not work for another, and that's totally okay. Joining a support group can be a game-changer. Surrounding yourself with like-minded moms gives you a platform to share, learn, and grow.

There's a wealth of collective wisdom in these groups that can guide you through those tricky phases. Breastfeeding is about more than just nourishment; it's about the bond, the silent conversations, and those moments of pure love. Sure, there might be hiccups along the way – but with the right guidance and mindset, they're just stepping stones to mastering the art. Your breastfeeding journey is your story, written by you and your little one. It's a chapter of growth, learning, and tons of love.

Dive in with an open heart and mind, and you'll find your way.

BREAST MILK AMOUNT DEPENDS ON BREAST SIZE

The volume of glandular tissue is pretty much the same for all women. This means that even with a "zero" breast size, there'll be enough milk for feeding. From the early days of pregnancy, thanks to a cocktail of hormones, your milk glands gear up for breastfeeding. They can swell up by 2-3 sizes. So, your starting breast size doesn't affect the milk quantity at all! However, the storage capacity of each woman's breast is different.

Let's visualise it.

Picture this: three people in front of bowls of porridge. Everyone has the same-sized bowl — that represents our daily milk volume. But the spoons they get are different: one has a ladle, another a regular spoon, and the third gets a teaspoon.

The spoons represent the storage capacity of our breasts. It's unrealistic to expect the teaspoon holder to empty their bowl in the same number of scoops as the ladle user. They'll still finish it; they'll just have to scoop more often. Breastfeeding is as natural as it gets, but it's also unique to every mom and baby duo. Sure, some moms might seem to fill up faster and need fewer feeding sessions, while others might be offering their breast more frequently.

And guess what? Both are perfectly normal. It's all about finding your own rhythm and not comparing your journey to anyone else's. We often hear the saying, "trust your body," and it couldn't be more accurate in this scenario. Your body knows what it's doing. Even if you're frequently feeding, it's just your body's way of ensuring your little one gets all they need. Over time, you'll notice patterns, and the two of you will sync up.

It's a dance, with its own tempo and unique steps.

THE LITTLE ONE GETS SO LITTLE COLOSTRUM, MAYBE THEY NEED SOMETHING EXTRA

The World Health Organization (or WHO if you're into the whole brevity thing) is like, "Hey, for newborns, let's stick to breast milk." That is, unless there's some legit medical reason to deviate. Little one's system? Totally not made for anything other than that liquid gold called colostrum and milk.

Colostrum? It's like nature's own special shake and it's been brewing in mom's diner for months before the baby's grand entrance. It's packed with just about every nutrient and essential thingy that your tiny human needs for the first 2-3 days of life. On day one, your baby's tummy is tiny – think 5-6 ml, about the size of a cherry, and isn't really ready for anything more than a few drops. Especially considering colostrum is kinda like a super-concentrated power smoothie. Fast forward to day three, and that tummy's grown to the size of a walnut, holding about 22-27 ml. Right around then, it's time for the transition milk to make its debut.

So, how do you know there's enough colostrum for your baby? A few signs:
- On day one, your baby's taking 1-2 pee breaks, by day two, it's 2-3 times, and this continues till day 14;
- The pee? Crystal clear and not stinky at all;
- By days two to three, the baby's poop game shifts from tar-like black (meconium) to greenish and then onto yellowish with some bits;
- After day four, expect about three diaper blowouts a day.

Moms, heads up: the more you get the baby on the breast, the quicker your body goes from colostrum mode to milk mode. So, keep an eye on the clock. Try not to let more than 2 hours pass between feeds during the day, and whenever you can, offer both sides during a single feed.

Your baby and your breasts will thank you!

YOU'LL WASTE YOUR MILK IF YOU DON'T PUMP OUT THE LEFTOVERS AFTER FEEDING

When feeding your baby on demand, mom's body pretty much ensures there's the right amount of milk. It's kind of like nature's own delivery system. So, when should you actually think about pumping?

1. If your little one loses more than 10% of their birth weight or struggles with sucking and weight gain.

2. When the doc suggests phototherapy.

3. For those special care plans for babies born a tad on the lighter side.

4. Got a super sleepy baby? And it's a task to wake them up, especially if they're out like a light for more than 2-3 hours.

5. If you're having a hard time pumping that first milk or colostrum, formula might be on the cards. But hey, keep up with that breast stimulation.

6. If the maternity ward has this thing where mom and baby get some time apart, or if delivery had its share of challenges, like a C-section.

7. If after feeding, one breast feels a bit too full, maybe pump just enough to feel better.

Just a heads up: Going all out with the pumping might cause you to produce too much milk. If baby's not up for all that milk, it could hang around in the breast, which isn't great and might lead to some issues.

Best to keep things balanced!

BREASTFEEDING WITH FLAT, LET ALONE INVERTED, NIPPLES IS A NO-GO

Babies aren't just latching onto the nipple. They grab a whole "chunk" of the breast, with the nipple just being the target. Wondering if you have inverted nipples? Press around it, both above and below:
- Pops out? It´s not inverted.
- Goes in? It's inverted.

During pregnancy, many women's nipples tend to become more protruding. And once your baby gets to work, they'll stretch even further. Inverted nipples provide less stimulation since they don't really poke out. But, when your baby suckles, they create a vacuum that can pull the nipple out.

However, two things:
- It might feel a tad weird.
- The baby needs to latch and start sucking for this magic to happen.

Tips for Breastfeeding Moms:
- Only offer the breast when your baby has their mouth wide open. This ensures a proper latch, capturing both the nipple and some areola.
- Give your nipples a little pre-game pep talk. Use a breast pump or some self-massage techniques. Basically, pinch with your thumb and index finger and pull forward.
- Express a bit of milk before feeding. It makes your breast softer and more yielding.
- Skin-to-skin is the way to go when feeding. It boosts the baby's natural instincts and strengthens the bond.
- Milk dribbles during feeds? Wipe it off with a clean cloth or tissue. Helps the baby maintain a good grip.

If you've tried all the DIY solutions and things still aren't clicking, seek advice from a breastfeeding expert. They've got your back!

YOU GOTTA BEAR THE PAIN AND WAIT FOR YOUR NIPPLES TO TOUGHEN UP

Yeah, it might sting a bit. This can go on for 2-3 weeks, and in rare cases, up to 3-6 months. Here's why some moms might get cracks and sores:
• Maybe you're still figuring out how to feed the little one comfortably and painlessly. Even a quick 5-minute feed every 3 hours can lead to sores, and then, yep, cracks.
• Washing your breasts before every feed and then using alcohol-based solutions? If you do, you're washing away the protective layer on the areola and drying out the skin.
• Maybe the baby isn't latching correctly.
• Baby could have a short tongue tie.
• Or, it could be a fungal or bacterial infection.

Here's what you can do:
• Find a comfy position for feeding – you'll be doing a lot of it in the first months!
• Keep an eye on the baby's latch and fix it if needed.
• If it hurts, don't just endure. Maybe try hand-expressing for a bit.
• Skip washing your breasts all the time.
• Let them breathe – literally! Air baths can help.
• After feeding, apply ointments with lanolin.
• Check if your baby has a tongue tie.
• Maybe use the breast pump a little less.
• Keep baby away from bottles and pacifiers. If you need to supplement, try using a syringe, cup, or spoon.

Breastfeeding ain't always easy, but with a bit of know-how, you can make it work for you

MYTH #8
STRESS CAN MAKE YOUR MILK DISAPPEAR

Lactation hinges on two key hormones: prolactin and oxytocin. Prolactin: Responsible for milk production. Good news? Your emotional state doesn't impact this guy.

Tips for maximizing prolactin's function:
- Ensure frequent breastfeeding sessions.
- Night-time feedings are crucial, especially between 3 to 8 AM when prolactin production peaks.
- Proper latching ensures optimal milk supply.

Oxytocin: This one handles the release of milk from the breast. It promotes contraction of muscle cells surrounding the mammary glands, facilitating milk flow. Here's the catch: its level is influenced by a mother's psychological state. If a mother is under significant stress or experiencing negative emotions, unwanted guests like cortisol and adrenaline spike, hindering oxytocin's function.

The result? Milk release becomes challenging. It can be hard for the baby to get any milk, and even manual expression or pumps might not yield much. Bigger Concerns: Not only could you face decreased milk supply, but there's also the potential of recurrent lactation blockages.

Facing Milk Flow Issues? It's time to focus on relaxation and positive reinforcements:
- When expressing, think about your baby; maybe even smell their clothing or gaze at their photos.
- Herbal teas with calming properties can be beneficial.
- Gentle shoulder massages might ease tension.
- Engage in calm conversations.
- Take a moment in a warm bath.

MYTH #9
"I'M JUST NOT MEANT TO PRODUCE MILK"

A genuine milk deficiency is experienced by only about 2-3% of mothers. The primary reasons could be severe hormonal imbalances. With certain hormonal conditions, it's challenging to conceive and carry a pregnancy to term. HOWEVER, many moms, even with such conditions, can still partially breastfeed their child.

"NO ONE IN MY FAMILY BREASTFED FOR MORE THAN A MONTH, AND I WAS ONLY BREASTFED FOR THREE WEEKS, ETC."

This belief is typically held by women who have previously had an unsuccessful breastfeeding experience. Or such notions creep in after talking to more "experienced" relatives. And from them come the age-old advice: feeding by the clock, supplementing with water/formula, or resorting to pacifiers. Following such "tips" can genuinely reduce milk production.

And the "I'm not meant to produce milk" mindset gets reaffirmed (just like grandma used to say, right?). Before concluding that you're "not cut out for breastfeeding" and giving up on it, it's essential to identify and rectify any breastfeeding mistakes. Lacking knowledge and confidence? Reach out for support from a lactation consultant or experienced breastfeeding moms who've had success.

With the right support, it's possible to rewrite your "hereditary" narrative.

BREASTFEEDING RUINS THE SHAPE OF THE BREAST AND BODY

Starting from pregnancy, the shape of the breasts doesn't return to its pre-pregnancy state. Interestingly, after extended breastfeeding, breasts can maintain a better shape than if one hadn't breastfed at all.

As for the body shape: when you breastfeed, you lose weight! That's a little bonus from nature. Producing milk burns around 500-700 calories, and many women start shedding pounds after six months of breastfeeding.

WHAT ACTUALLY RUINS THE BODY SHAPE:
• Eating more under the misconception of "eating for two" to ensure there's "enough milk" and consuming more fatty foods so the milk is "richer" (more on this later).
• Finishing the leftovers of your child.

If you stop breastfeeding but retain the habit of overeating, that's when you can actually gain weigh

TO PRODUCE MORE MILK, YOU SHOULD "FEAST" ON HIGH-CALORIE FOODS AND DRINK TEA WITH MILK

Remember, milk production is a hormonal process. The amount of milk is produced regardless of how many times a mother has eaten during the day. She can survive on just black bread and water and still produce quality milk. However, in this case, her body will work at its own expense to produce good milk for the baby in the required quantity.

The mother's body uses an additional 700 kcal daily to produce milk. 500 of these come from the food she consumes. Another 200 kcal comes from the fat stores accumulated during pregnancy.

NUTRITION IS NEEDED NOT FOR THE MILK, BUT TO MAINTAIN THE MOTHER'S VITAL ENERGY.

For the production of milk with all the necessary elements, the mother needs to eat a diverse diet and only when she's hungry.

The same goes for water and other beverages. Drinking too much can be more of a detriment to breastfeeding than a benefit.
- "Excess" water puts a strain on a woman's excretory system.
- It can lead to breast engorgement or lactostasis (milk stasis).
- The body might activate its defence mechanisms and start suppressing lactation.

FLUIDS DO AFFECT LACTATION, but not the amount of milk. Instead, they influence the speed of its ejection from the breast. Any hot liquid consumed 10-15 minutes before feeding stimulates the release of oxytocin, consequently causing a milk ejection reflex.

The belief in the magical properties of tea with milk, especially if condensed, is particularly popular.

CONSIDER:
• Of all foreign proteins to the human body, cow's milk protein (CMP) most often causes allergic reactions.
• The quantity of a woman's breast milk doesn't change whether you drink cow's milk or not. After all, no mammal drinks another mammal's milk to produce its own.

It's surprising that in a world where this myth exists, there's a counteracting myth.

A BREASTFEEDING MOTHER MUST FOLLOW A STRICT DIET

Pregnancy, childbirth, and breastfeeding are natural physiological processes. Their success is not linked to any particular strict diet. No mammal changes its diet after giving birth!

Food should be customary. It's preferable not to include exotic foods that are not typical for one's "native" climate zone. A nursing mother might develop unique food cravings, and they should be satisfied just like the cravings of a pregnant woman.

However, the primary principle is that food should be diverse, contain as many natural products as possible, and have minimal chemicals.

And what about the foods that cause the baby to get bloated? Such products like cabbage, cucumbers, black bread, beans, etc., are often blacklisted.

REALITY: Milk is synthesized from components of blood and lymph, not the contents of the mother's stomach. Only artificial additives, e.g., chemical colorants or medicines, enter breast milk unchanged. Even then, the concentration of some is comparable to their levels in the mother's blood, while others are even lower. No cabbage gets into the milk, so it can't cause bloating.

In half of the cases, an unbiased assessment (especially if the nursing mother tries to eat the same "dangerous" product a week later) shows that the baby reacted to something else, such as a change in the weather. In other cases, there's an individual reaction to a product, especially in the mother. Not everyone digests food equally well. Some products cause heartburn, flatulence, or have a laxative or binding effect on the mother. Depending on the intensity of the reaction, there can be changes in the mother's blood, some of which may reflect in the milk's composition. In such cases, the baby's reaction to these changes is possible but not guaranteed.

FACTORS THAT CAN AFFECT THE BABY'S MOOD:
- Retrograde Mercury
- Badly smelling products affecting the taste of milk? This usually refers to onions, garlic, radishes, broccoli, and strongly scented spices.
- Weather
- Other factors
- The mother's individual reaction

Products that affect the taste and smell of milk might exist. However, they don't impact a child's appetite or the frequency of breastfeeding. An experiment in England with a list of twenty "suspicious" products showed that only two products affected the volume of milk the baby consumed. When mothers consumed garlic, babies actually consumed more milk. Apparently, they liked the strong smell of garlic!

A special diet is only necessary when the mother has a severe allergy, or her diet isn't well-rounded. If you suffer from food allergies, you will need to pay more attention to your diet.

MY CHILD DEMANDS A PACIFIER

Children are ALWAYS conditioned to a pacifier. Usually, the first time a child gets a pacifier is when he shows restlessness, and the mother doesn't know how to calm him down. To soothe, a child needs to suckle on the breast. If they don't get the breast, they'll have to suckle on whatever else is provided.

PROS OF A PACIFIER:
- Pacifiers can be a quick way to calm a fussy baby, especially during situations where breastfeeding might not be immediately possible.
- Some studies suggest that using a pacifier during sleep can reduce the risk of sudden infant death syndrome (SIDS).

CONS OF A PACIFIER:
- Excessive use of a pacifier might lead to missed breastfeeding sessions, which in rare cases could contribute to milk stasis.
- Transitioning between a breast and a pacifier might confuse some babies due to the different sucking mechanisms.
- Pacifiers can be a source of potential infection if not kept clean, especially when dropped frequently.
- Over-reliance on pacifiers might, in some cases, impact the development of the jaw and teeth, even if using an orthodontic pacifier.
- There's a possibility, though not conclusive, that prolonged pacifier use can lead to minor speech delays.

IF A CHILD OFTEN ASKS FOR THE BREAST, IT MEANS THEY'RE HUNGRY AND NOT GETTING ENOUGH MILK

There are several reasons why a child might ask to be breastfed, and it's not always just about hunger.

NEED FOR MOTHER'S CONTACT:

For the first three months after birth, newborns have an inherent need for regular contact with their mother. This is primarily because the baby needs to feel safe and protected. Their entire focus is on establishing and maintaining this vital connection.

GROWING BODY:

During the first month after birth, breastfeeding every hour is physiologically normal. As they grow, the frequency reduces. The stomach of a newborn is designed to receive milk in frequent, small amounts. It's incapable of holding 150-200 ml of milk at once. Hence, infants in their first few months ask for the breast up to 15-20 times a day, including multiple times at night.

PAIN RELIEF:

Newborns can experience pain due to various reasons: intestinal colic, fever, or teething. Regular breastfeeding not only nourishes them but also soothes their nervous system and alleviates pain.

DESIRE TO BE SOOTHED:

Babies can feel anxious too. And who's the best at comforting them? The mother. Infants often seek the comfort of their mother's breast during the early months, and it's entirely normal.

GROWTH SPURTS:

Newborns go through phases of rapid growth. During these growth spurts, they need more nutrients than usual. In such situations, mothers should not deny breastfeeding. These growth phases typically last no more than four days.

WE CAN DETERMINE IF A BABY HAS ENOUGH MILK BY DOING A "CONTROL FEEDING."

A baby fed on demand often extracts varying amounts of milk. It could be 5 ml in one feeding, 50 ml the next, and 150 ml in another. The newborn's body is adapted to intake small portions of milk frequently. Therefore, even if fed 6-7 times a day, an infant typically extracts small milk portions, not 6 servings of 120 ml each. Hence, there might be cases of underfeeding and weight loss.

THERE ARE TWO MAIN WAYS TO ASSESS IF A BABY IS GETTING ENOUGH MILK:

Wet Diaper Test: Remove the baby's diapers and count the number of urinations in a day. If there are 10-12, it indicates sufficient milk intake. However, if there are only 6-8, you might need to increase the feeding frequency.

Weekly Weight Gain: For babies older than 7 days, a weekly weight gain ranging from 125 grams to 500 grams is a good sign. It's recommended to weigh the baby no more than once a week!

YOU NEED TO "STORE" MILK FOR BREASTFEEDING

The breast is never truly "empty." In response to a baby's suckling, milk is constantly being produced. However, if a mother waits for the breast to fill up, she gradually reduces the amount of milk being produced over time, causing the milk to "burn," as some might say.

If the baby skips a feeding, they don't "order" food for the next meal because they haven't stimulated prolactin production.

If milk isn't expressed, an inhibitory hormone in the breast signals the brain that the milk is rarely used and that as much isn't needed, leading to the risk of lactostasis.

THE MORE OFTEN A MOTHER NURSES HER BABY, THE MORE MILK SHE PRODUCES.

YOU MUST FEED YOUR BABY ON A SCHEDULE; OTHERWISE, THEY WILL OVEREAT AND RISK BECOMING OBESE

This belief might apply to formula-fed babies since the formula's composition and energy content remain constant.

However, breastfeeding is a different ball game:

Adaptive: Breast milk changes to meet the baby's needs.

Digestive-friendly: Contains enzymes like lipase that aid digestion without overburdening the baby's system.

Quick Digestion: Breast milk coagulates swiftly in the stomach, moving to the intestines for digestion and absorption within 40 minutes.

A newborn's stomach is designed to receive frequent small amounts of milk. Holding 150-200 ml at once is just not feasible. Hence, infants often feed up to 15-20 times a day, including several times at night.

Typically, a baby establishes its feeding rhythm by 2-3 months of age.

MYTH #18
AFTER FEEDING, YOU SHOULD
HOLD THE BABY UPRIGHT

It's typically formula-fed babies that need to be held upright to prevent the 120g of formula from spilling.

For breastfed babies who feed on demand and consume smaller amounts of mother's milk, there's no need to hold them upright. Such infants spend most of their time lying on their side. It's normal for a baby to spit up about 2-3 tablespoons after each feeding and the esophageal sphincter to release once in a forceful manner.

Moreover, the cardiac sphincter of the stomach needs exercise. Its development is somewhat underdeveloped to allow both milk and air to be released with ease. This action, in turn, helps train the sphincter, and the training occurs primarily when the baby is lying down.

NIGHT IS FOR SLEEP

For newborns, it's normal to have one prolonged sleep per day that lasts 4-5 hours. During the rest of the day, they might sleep in intervals ranging from 20 minutes to 1.5-2 hours, and this is also considered normal.

IF A BABY SLEEPS TOO MUCH AND DOESN'T GAIN WEIGHT WELL, OFFER THE BREAST MORE OFTEN. For infants, it's completely natural to wake up several times during the night because:

The physiology of an infant is such that their sleep cycle lasts about 40 minutes. Sleep consists of two phases: light sleep and deep sleep. Since babies aren't fully developed at birth, they don't naturally transition from one cycle to the next. During light sleep, they need assistance to transition into the next cycle. This help can come in the form of breastfeeding, rocking, shushing, or patting.

Nighttime nursing stimulates the mother's prolactin levels, ensuring a decent milk supply during the day.

The baby may be experiencing stress, anxiety, teething, a fever, or a growth spurt. In all these situations, breastfeeding can be soothing and comforting.

Expecting a child to sleep through the night like an adult is unrealistic until they are around 1-2 years old with proper approach to the sleep schedule.

FEEDING ON DEMAND IS A NIGHTMARE! IT'S IMPOSSIBLE TO SIT AND FEED THE BABY ALL DAY LONG!

With properly organized breastfeeding, the mother can rest! She lies down, relaxed, embraces the baby, and the baby nurses. During the first 1-1.5 months after birth, when the baby latches on sporadically, without a clear routine, and nurses frequently and for extended periods, the mother can feel good only if the breastfeeding is organized correctly.

The mother should be comfortable nursing in various positions like standing, lying down, sitting, and even moving.

IT'S BEST TO KEEP A BABY AT THE BREAST FOR NO LONGER THAN 15 MINUTES

In the first week of life, a newborn might indeed latch relatively infrequently – 7-8 times a day. However, by the second week, the intervals between feedings often decrease. When awake, the baby might ask for breastmilk up to four times in an hour, meaning every 15 minutes! Typically, a baby fed on demand will latch around 12 or more times a day in the first month, often between 16-20 times.

If you think that a baby only shows a desire to feed by crying, that's not the case. Here's a list of more subtle signs of hunger:

- Moving hands during sleep and clenching fists.
- Waking up, but not yet crying.
- Opening the mouth and sticking out the tongue.
- Pulling things like swaddling cloth or their own hand to their mouth, sucking on the mother's hand when held in a cradle position, or trying to suck the mother's thumb.
- Making sounds as if "talking."
- Movement of the eyes during rapid sleep; the baby might need to latch upon waking.
- Turning the head during sleep or while awake.

Regrettably, in many cases, when a baby begins to demand the breast more frequently, mothers may assume the child is starving and introduce supplementary feeding. Or they might artificially increase the intervals between feedings.

However, there's a potential pitfall for both mother and baby: insufficient breast stimulation can result in decreased milk production. The concept of feeding on demand does not entertain the replacement of breastfeeding with a pacifier or bottle.

YOU NEED TO "STORE" MILK FOR BREASTFEEDING

Feedings longer than 10 minutes assist the baby in achieving growth, weight gain, brain development, and the maturation of the gastrointestinal tract. They also normalize digestive processes and contribute to building a strong immune system. When a baby stays at the breast for an extended period, they receive what is often referred to as the "hindmilk," which is richer in fats.

SHORTER LATCHINGS SERVE TO:
• Quench thirst since breast milk is composed of approximately 90% water.
• Reduce anxiety.
• Ensure the regular functioning of the nervous system during times of overload.

BABIES ENJOY SAVORING the taste and often fall asleep while sucking. However, if one tries to remove the breast prematurely, they can quickly wake up and resume sucking. As a result, a feeding session might last 30-40 minutes, and sometimes even longer.

MYTH #23
YOU MUST ALWAYS GIVE WATER TO A NEWBORN BECAUSE MILK IS FOOD

Breast milk consists of approximately 90% water (and this particular water is best assimilated by the baby). Supplementing a baby with additional water can disrupt the balance between fluid intake and output, as well as increase the load on the kidneys. In the first months of life, a baby's ability to excrete fluid is about ten times less than that of an adult.

Even in hot weather, it's essential to offer the breast to the baby. Milk is a physiological fluid containing an optimal concentration of salts and minerals. Furthermore, in a baby's brain, the centers for satiety and thirst quenching are so closely linked that the intake of water is perceived as food consumption. When you supplement your baby with additional liquids, consider that they may likely consume less milk as they "process" the water or infant tea.

THE BABY IS NOT GETTING ENOUGH NUTRIENTS; COMPLEMENTARY FEEDING SHOULD START AT FOUR MONTHS

It makes sense to introduce complementary foods no earlier than at six months of age. By this age, the baby's immune system is stronger, and the digestive system is ready. However, when starting with complementary foods, it's essential not to abandon breastfeeding. Breast milk remains the primary source of nutrition for the baby during the first and second years of life. Complementary foods do not replace breast milk; they only supplement it. Introducing complementary foods too early might have several adverse effects:

• It could influence the quantity of breast milk: the baby might breastfeed less frequently, causing the milk production to decrease. Complementary foods should not interfere with breastfeeding;
• Early complementary feeding can trigger allergic reactions;
• Due to an underdeveloped digestive system, there's a risk of upsetting the baby's stomach and intestines.

WHEN YOU HAVE BREAST ENGORGEMENT, YOU SHOULD PRESS THE BREAST AS HARD AS POSSIBLE

Breast engorgement usually subsides within 12-48 hours after the onset of milk production. Here are some ways to prevent and deal with it:

1. Breastfeed Early and Often: Feed as soon as possible and frequently. Avoid using substitutes. Try to feed the baby as soon after birth as you can. Attach the baby to the breast at least ten times a day. Switch feeding positions (e.g., cradle, from under the arm, lying down).
2. Ensure Proper Latching: Ensure the baby latches on correctly. Feed whenever the baby indicates a desire to breastfeed.
3. Awaken the Baby for Feeding: If the baby sleeps for more than 2-3 hours consecutively during the day or more than 4 hours at night, wake him/her up for feeding.
4. Let the Baby Nurse Fully: Allow the baby to nurse on one breast as long as they want. Typically, babies will either fall asleep or release the breast when satiated.
5. Don't Limit Nursing Time: Don't limit the nursing time on one breast to a specific number of minutes.
6. Express Milk: If the baby isn't nursing or isn't nursing well, express milk either by hand or with a breast pump as frequently as if the baby were nursing. It's generally recommended to express milk at least 8 times a day (every 2-3 hours from both breasts).
7. Hydrate: Drink according to thirst.

ADVICE AND WARNINGS:
• Do not express through pain or turn to professionals who suggest you should express with unbearable pain, leaving bruises and dents on the swollen breast. This could lead to blockages and mastitis.
• Avoid using a breast pump on an engorged breast, as it could lead to further swelling and possibly mastitis.
• Don't limit your water intake hoping to reduce milk production. Reduced water intake can lead to edema.
• Don't give the baby formula thinking he/she is "hungry." The volume of formula consumed does not equate to breast milk volume.

• Feed even if one breast is sore. Avoiding it can exacerbate the situation.

• Don't take anti-lactation pills. Blocked milk ducts and the hormone prolactin are two different things, with potential severe side effects.

• Don't apply heat to the breast. Inflammation around a blocked duct can become a site for microbial growth, leading to infectious mastitis or an abscess.

• Do not let the husband express the milk. Adults have different techniques, and there's a risk of introducing infections.

WHEN TO SEE A DOCTOR:

• If engorgement does not resolve despite trying the above measures.

• If you experience symptoms of mastitis: a temperature above 38.5°C, red/painful/swollen breasts, chills, or flu-like symptoms.

• If the baby cannot latch onto the breast.

• If the baby has fewer wet and soiled diapers than usual.

ABOUT THE AUTHOR

Meet Lyria Haven: a mom of five who can expertly balance a toddler on one hip and a latte on the other. With years of hands-on experience and countless "I've been there" moments, Lyria has earned her unofficial PhD in the School of Real-Life Parenting. When she's not decoding toddler gibberish or hunting for lost toys, she's penning down her candid and research-backed insights about pregnancy and motherhood. Lyria´s books artfully combine hilariously honest anecdotes with proven advice, making them a must-read for any parent seeking both laughter and guidance. If you've ever found yourself wondering if that stain is chocolate or... something else, or needed solid advice amidst the chaos, Lyria's your gal. She may be winging some of it (aren't we all?), but she's got the creds and the lived experience to back it up!

www.ingramcontent.com/pod-product-compliance
Lightning Source LLC
Chambersburg PA
CBHW070754260726
48660CB00007B/3122